RZ LR

Enfield

GW00340756

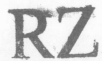

Your name is OLGA

JOSEP M. ESPINÁS

TRANSLATED BY
PAMELA WALEY

FOREWORD BY
CLAIRE RAYNER

UNWIN HYMAN
London   Sydney   Wellington

Originally published in Catalan under the title *El teu nom és Olga* by Edicions La Campana, Barcelona.

First published in English in Great Britain by the Trade Division of Unwin Hyman Limited, 1989.

UNWIN HYMAN LIMITED
15–17 Broadwick Street
London W1V 1FP

Allen & Unwin Australia Pty Ltd
8 Napier Street, North Sydney, NSW 2060, Australia

Allen & Unwin New Zealand Pty Ltd with the
Port Nicholson Press, Compusales Building, 75 Ghuznee Street,
Wellington, New Zealand

British Library Cataloguing in Publication Data

Espinas, Josep M.
Your name is Olga.
1. Down's syndrome children. Care –
Personal observations
I. Title
362.3

ISBN 0-04-440404-2

Phototypeset by Computape (Pickering) Ltd, North Yorkshire
Printed in Great Britain by Biddles Ltd, Guildford

You call her mongol
We call her Down's child
Her friends call her by her name*

* Text of a poster of the
Down's Syndrome Association

CONTENTS

INTRODUCTION
BY CLAIRE RAYNER

In an ideal world all children would be born well and beautiful with all the promise of a completely capable adult future carried safely in their new small hands. But this is the real world and that means that some babies are born less than healthy, though still beautiful (I never yet saw a really ugly baby, did you?) and with their potential for the future deeply damaged.

Among those damaged babies are those who are born with the condition labelled Down's Syndrome. The range of symptoms these babies show is very wide. The abilities they have are very varied. Their hopes for a capable future are as different as their families are. But they are all babies, and all important to the parents who bore them and the people who look after them.

This book is therefore not about all babies with Down's Syndrome. Just about one of them. Olga is the daughter of a well respected and established Spanish author and he has written these letters to her, because, as he says himself in these pages, he realized that his relationship with his special daughter was one he ought to share with other Down's children's parents, other children with the problems and perhaps above all with those who have never been touched by the problems it causes, so that they will understand.

It's a lovely book, in every sense of the word. Lovely to read and filled with love. At one point in it Olga's father says, "Like any other child, a Down's constructs his or her character with the mysterious but certain materials of genetic inheritance and the no less subtle but unquestionable materials provided by his or her environment. The Down's child isn't a finished product but a human being who can change and develop through the influences he or she receives." And Olga is one of the world's lucky ones. It is clear from these letters that she has received superb influences in making the best of the hand she was dealt with at birth.

Most importantly, she has been loved and

cared for by a family that learned very early that there was no guilt on them for Olga's situation. In a letter headed "I don't want to know why" Olga's father writes, "No one is to blame for your problem, Olga, and on this point the parents of children like you have to put out of their minds from the very start any suspicion of doubt or anxiety. This doesn't always happen, unfortunately. I know some very sad cases of a father or mother who has sought to extricate themselves from the reality that was burdening them with accusations or suspicion against the other. You and others like you, Olga, do something that is really very hard: you put adults to the test, and sometimes it is evident that the adults are not very adult." And that is almost the most important message in the book.

But not quite. There are others. Such as the fact that learning and developing for all of us, and not just for Down's children, can and does go on well into adult life. Olga is now very much an adult, at thirty-two, but still learning, still finding new abilities. And it is clear her father is too.

And there is another important message; which is that all children, be they handicapped or able-bodied, are different. Olga differs from other children in the same way that able-bodied children differ from each other. She is her own person, her own character and her degree of handicap does not alter that, even if it does, for the less perceptive, mask it.

And yet another vital message; which is that parents do for their children what they want to do and not because they ought to. To quote again: "One of the great problems of emotional relationships is that they are relationships that require a certain repayment. It happens between married couples, between friends, and between parents and children. Nowadays there are still many mothers and fathers who persist in the traditional requirement that children should show gratitude for everything their parents have done for them. (A nuance: they don't have to be grateful at all, but they have to show it.) And they have to show it not in the way that seems logical to the child, but in the way the parents require it. There is always the danger that the understandable desire to be repaid may be converted into moral blackmail. 'After all we've done for you . . .'"

Olga's father has avoided that trap and, in telling us of it, helps to point it out so that we may avoid it too. And he has done more in this book; he has offered insights that we can all share. "To have a subnormal child," he says, "is not an experience to be desired. But I should be the undesirable one if over the years I had not come to realize that you and I, Olga, have both been enriched by our mutual love and also by our mutual training – and yes, I have learnt from you too." Olga couldn't have a better accolade.

Dear Reader

This is a book I had to write. I wrote it straight off, perhaps because that was the only way to avoid having time for self-criticism, doubts, reflection and, in short, prudence, which might have made me leave it unwritten.

It's possible that not everything I say in it – about Olga, my Down's Syndrome daughter, about myself, other people and life – is absolutely true, but it is what I think and what I feel. I know that these pages are therefore easily vulnerable, as are all public confessions.

Over the years I have become increasingly convinced that the relationship between Olga and myself is not a strictly private matter, and certainly my profession as a writer has urged me to run the risk of being too bold. Risk is often the friend that helps us to make friends, and I would like all the Olgas in the world to have more of those every day.

So I had to write these pages, and I should have regretted not doing it in time because I think that if there is anything of value in this book it is the love of life.

JME

1 WE HAD NEVER IMAGINED . . .

Dear Olga

We had never imagined that you might not be "normal", as they call it.

Indeed, to tell the truth, we hadn't imagined anything; we had never thought of you in any concrete way. We were going to have a boy or a girl, and that was it. At that time, thirty-one years ago, it wasn't possible to know the sex of a child before birth, and parents used to choose names in advance, a boy's name and a girl's name so as not to be taken by surprise.

It's strange, but I don't remember what name we had thought of for you if you had been a boy.

If we had one, we've forgotten it. Do you know, Olga, how many unnecessary worries in this life you have helped us to forget?

No, we never imagined that we might have a daughter like you.

Nowadays perhaps more people are aware of the possibility because people like you are discussed more often, and go about in public more and live longer, and gradually your presence is becoming more accepted: for parents today the appearance of a "mongol" child may be worrying, but in 1954 it was almost unthinkable.

Two years before you existed someone asked me to visit the centre founded by Dr Jeroni de Moragas, a wonderful teacher who cared for children like you. At that time I was writing for a periodical, *Destino*, and it was thought that if I wrote a few lines on the school it might be of use to it and consequently to the Moragas family, who seemed to be going through a difficult time in the post-war years. When I left their house in Barcelona it was with a heavy heart, I must admit, and perhaps because of that I have always understood those strangers who can't help an instinctive gesture of withdrawal when they come across people like you. I find this absolutely natural, and at the same time I think that nature has been very compassionate towards you in making you unaware of it.

Then, in July 1952, Jeroni de Moragas wrote me a letter, which I kept, and I couldn't foresee then how much it was to mean to me:

Dear friend, thank you, thank you many times, for your successful article, exact, clear and precise, which was just what was wanted. It has been of great service to me. I am especially grateful for the apt concept, which had never occurred to me, of *"diminished* childhood"*. It conveys all that needs to be said, with all possible love. I shall use it myself from now on.

My friend Moragas – who would have been your friend too, Olga, because you've had the good fortune to have many friends (we'll discuss those another day) – saw in the idea of "mental diminishment" an expression of love, because in those days "abnormal" (and, before that, "subnormal") sounded like a slap in the face. But now it could be discussed in terms of a word that conveyed "all that needs to be said, with all possible love". I've learnt that in this case, and surely in other cases, great love makes you say things with the right word, or at least with a word that people can identify with the reality. In the course of time we won the right to present ourselves publicly as parents of subnormal children, and in using the word which others, through tactfulness, didn't dare to apply to our children in front of us I think we performed an act of affirmation of love.

Some people will call you "defective", Olga, but you mustn't let it bother you: it is true, but it isn't the whole truth. Others will call you "sub-normal", and we will accept that too, won't we, because there is no point in trying to conceal a reality by splitting hairs over what is "normal" and what is "subnormal". If they think "mongol", they are making another approxi-mation, also a valid one, and if they define you as a Down's Syndrome case the tone is more neutral but it comes to the same thing.

You see, Olga, I know what you *are*, and no label or diagnosis which tries to explain you and all those who are like you can come anywhere near describing what that is.

You know it too, and when you knock at the door of my study, when I've shut myself away to do some writing, to tell me that dinner is ready or that I'm wanted on the phone, you say it aloud: "It's me, Olga."

It's me. We are all "me", but what happens is that we don't fully understand it because we only use "me" to talk about ourselves. Grammar has taught us to distinguish: I, you, he, she, we, they. In other words, other people are not "me".

We need to know this rule of grammar in

order to speak properly, but to believe it as a truth is absolutely useless for thinking properly. We run the risk of thinking that we are the only genuine "me" when the truth is that every other person is also "me" to himself and the rest of us are his "you" or his "he" or "she".

It was you, Olga, who most helped me to discover this, because you forced me – yes, indeed you did – to accept that I couldn't see you just as "you" or "she", as someone only related to me from outside myself, from a secondary or subordinate level.

I've had to think who you were, what your rights were, that you weren't like one of those many people whom we are used to seeing only as extras, as satellite figures in the scenario of our lives. I've had to free myself from my "me" vision of the world and understand that you too are a centre in human life, just as much a "me" – just as much the leading figure, the unique protagonist in your world – as any other person can be in his.

My world is wider. That is the only difference, and certainly an insignificant difference for anyone who hasn't a sick "me", an inflated "me". Does a blade of grass not have a "me" because it isn't an oak-tree?

You don't know this, but every time you come and say "It's me" you are not only putting yourself precisely in your place but also making me realize mine – I am your "you" – and, moreover, you are putting everything else in the world in its place.

2 BEING MORE USEFUL

Dear Olga

I was saying that we had never imagined that
you might not be normal, but the truth is that we
didn't suspect it even after you were born. We
couldn't foresee it, and we couldn't see it either.

We had no experience of such a thing. Probably the obstetrician saw it at once, but he didn't
say anything to us. Nobody told us what was
happening for a long time, many weeks, even
months, when it began to be only too obvious
that your reactions weren't the usual ones.

We must have behaved in such an ignorant
and innocent way that our relatives and the

paediatrician had to suffer considerably, and we are sorry now that we couldn't have done anything to help them. Finally Dr Renan, the paediatrician and a good man, told us one day that perhaps you wouldn't be able to study but that you could be a housewife . . . Only at that moment did our eyes begin to open. Why did he dare prophesy already that in some future time you wouldn't be good at school work . . . ?

With hindsight I think that that ambiguousness, that letting time pass so that we could develop and very gradually discover the truth for ourselves without a sudden verdict, was a good idea, and the typical "over-reaction to diagnosis" was minimal.

They didn't "label" you, dear Olga, and present you to us too quickly and irrevocably as a misfortune. We had time to learn to live with our worries, to realize that they required us to make special efforts, and when we finally learnt the truth you were already part of our normal life. I must say it because it's true: there was no drama. At home there was never any argument, no shouting and screaming, no despondency because of you, Olga. And I use the word "cause" and not "fault". Sometimes it seems to me strange that we never asked ourselves the exasperated question "why?". There's no point in asking ourselves "why did it happen to *us*?"

unless at the same time we ask "why did it happen to *you*?"; and asking ourselves those two questions at the same time the answer was of course pointless and instead was replaced by a calm acceptance of the hazards of life. So hazard united us.

Because you weren't born with an instinct for sucking, in order for you to survive we had to feed you, drop by drop. We put milk into a hypodermic syringe – without the needle – and held it between your motionless lips.

It must have done you good because you grew – and it did us good too. We had been landed with an unexpected responsibility, and young as we were we too had to take it gradually, drop by drop.

I don't think that I am a very patient person at all, and without you I should be still less so. We normal people have some natural qualities, Olga, which come to us easily, and other qualities which we can acquire or improve through the discomfort of an obligatory apprenticeship. We often say: "I'm no use at that" because something doesn't come easily to us at once. What we are actually saying without realizing it is: "I'm no use at trying to see if I'm any good at it."

Only in exceptional circumstances or under pressure which obliges us to decide between a risk and an extremely damaging defeat do we break away from our inertia and explore our possibilities. You do it too, Olga; you're as comfort-loving, as you say, as we are, and because of your "hurting" leg, when I'm walking along with you over uneven ground you want to hold my hand. But if we're staying at our country home at Solius, and you want to find out if the Cots family have arrived so that they can take you to church the next day in their car, you go off on your own, and you cross over irrigation ditches and climb up stairs without needing anyone to help. Sometimes I've watched you from a distance, and I know how difficult it is for you to make a certain step. But you've done it. You too are good at more things than you think. We can all do more things when there's no one to do them for us.

You taught us to do more things, and, conditioned by you, I discovered that they come naturally. You were the "exceptional circumstance" I mentioned, in which the two options were renunciation or commitment. You know that I have done some singing and that I write for newspapers and television, but you don't know that sometimes people have talked about my wish to serve. The results have been modest, but it's a fact that I undertook voluntary work. What they don't know is that it was you who aroused and fostered this wish. I owe it to you.

And to your example. Because when you grew up you showed that you have very strong will-power, and this impressed your teachers at the Boscana centre.

Since you came to do everything rather late it was a great effort for you to learn to walk. Those first, awkward steps were very important steps in another sense, towards your independence and your possibilities for social relationships. A few years later you had a very serious setback: some kind of infection destroyed the head of one of your hip-bones and the joint, and they had to operate on you. They dealt with it, but you were left with one leg shorter than the other. You were in bed for a long time, and I doubted whether you could learn all over again what had been so difficult for you when you had no such physical problem. But your will-power became "super-normal", and only you know how you managed to walk again, starting with a few slow steps, holding on to two chairs . . .

At school, in spite of your lame leg, you never let yourself be beaten by the exercises. I was very proud of you the day your teacher told me that you had explained to her: "I can't climb up there on my own like the others, but if you put your arm like this, you'll see what I can do . . ."

And that's an example to us all: to be able to ask for help but just the right and necessary amount of it to complement our own maximum effort.

We are sometimes too proud, Olga, and we don't ask for help, and sometimes we are too shameless or too spoiled and want other people to do what is really up to us.

It's very clear to you, though: you do all that you can, and you ask us to help you to do what is beyond your will-power.

And I can't describe my feelings when you say, so seriously, so conscientiously, "please".

3 NORMAL PARENTS

Dear Olga

It's so nice when you ask me "please" to do anything that it is my duty to do.

Being what you are, you've never made me feel that any duty was a nuisance; certainly not that of speaking out in public to defend the rights of people who are like you.

It all began one evening when a couple called Mr and Mrs Martínez de Foix came to see me at home. I didn't know them at all. I don't remember how the conversation started, but after a while they explained their position. They were the parents of a mentally retarded child and belonged to a recently formed group called ASPANIAS, the Association of Parents of Sub-normal Children and Adolescents. They had come to me, they said, because I wrote in the papers and could help them to make the exist-ence of the association more widely known and to make society more aware of a subject that was then practically taboo.

Their tact was exquisite because at no time did they drop any hint to make me suppose that they knew I was in the same position as them. Obviously they did know and it was because of this that they had come to see me, but their respect for my freedom of action was exemplary. In other words, they did it very well, and the proof is that I was soon talking to them about you, Olga, and I think that when I did so they felt much more at ease, as I did too.

From that day I became a member of ASPANIAS, and, although I play only a modest part, I've been helping for quite a long time. The rest of the committee were working much harder in practical ways, and generously gave their time and energy to unending negotiations which often ran up against an incredible lack of understanding on the part of the civil authorities and other bodies, and the more comprehensible reticence of parents of children like you. Because, Olga, you have to realize that people used to hide away such children, and we shouldn't now find fault with them for that, which would be unfair. What should I have done even now if I had lived in other circumstances, if I had been brought up differently or if I had another kind of temperament, if the Martínez de Foix had not got me involved or if you yourself had not been such a very agreeable person – you really are an extraordinarily nice and affectionate person, Olga – and aroused such feelings of solidarity?

But only a handful of parents – and there were many thousands of them – could accept the fact. Something had to be done to free them from mistaken feelings of shame – a social inheritance – of impotence and of having failed in life. The problem had to be aired, as they say, and brought out into the open, and to bring it out into the open we had to go out ourselves. If we didn't put in an appearance, how could we ask for anything?

Part of the task was entrusted to me because I could help by drawing up notices for the press and by accompanying them – because I was fairly well known – on visits to people. I found myself writing articles as a father, drawing attention to the lack of public interest in subnormal people, and also putting on the stage the first entertainment whose object, rather than making money, was to turn into news a subject too often ignored.

You must realize, Olga, that I didn't do this thinking of you, nor did my companions think of their own children. We could see clearly that it was too late to help resolve our own problems but that we had to work for future generations and set in train a movement to help those who would one day be parents of subnormal children, so that they would find themselves in a more favourable position from every point of view: medical attention, training centres within every-one's means, financial aid, social support . . .

We had started on a new song, which brought me much happiness, and a very bitter lesson. One day I received an anonymous letter, which I tore up at once but which I've always remembered. It said: "It seems incredible that with a mongol daughter you have the nerve and the insensitivity to appear, singing, in public." The unknown writer wanted to hurt me but only managed to reinforce what I felt (and ensure that I went on singing with an even stronger motive).

According to the anonymous writer, I should have become your victim, Olga . . . and by crip-pling myself as a person I would end up making you the victim of my frustration.

It has been obvious to me for a long time that

the first right of subnormal children is to have normal parents.

Normal means parents who accept their defective child as a human being who is a part of their life, not one who destroys it.

Normal means parents who understand that their relationship with their child has to be compatible with their natural relationship with the rest of the family, with friends, with everyone.

Normal means parents who don't collapse in the face of misfortune, but who know how to value the great and the small satisfactions which life also brings.

Normal means parents who don't enjoy castigating themselves through a perverted conscience.

Normal means parents who, instead of cherishing unhealthily the exceptionalness of their parenthood, cherish constructively their normalness as persons.

You and your friends, Olga, need parents who are capable of laughing, of being enthusiastic about plans, of going out to dances and to dinner with friends, of being happy so as to pass on to you happiness and not sadness, of being balanced so as to pass on to you comfort and not suffering, parents who are not perpetually thinking of you, because you need parents who are mentally and emotionally open and healthy.

More than other children, you need normal parents.

And ones who sing.

You enjoy singing a lot, Olga. If only you knew how happy it makes me to hear you sing!

So tell me this: if you sing, why shouldn't I?

4 INTELLECTUAL, MENTAL, PSYCHOLOGICAL

Dear Olga

You had a lovely time yesterday when we went to dinner with some new friends who live outside Barcelona.

You like making new friends – you said so – just as we do. You're glad that you have a lot of friends, as indeed you have. All our friends are your friends too, and we have to agree that we've been very fortunate. We are surrounded by understanding, affectionate, intelligent and tender-hearted people.

But if the relationship is such an easy one, it's because we've been fortunate with you. You are

the most tactful and best-mannered person I
know. If I were to say that you never get in the
way some people might think that you are
passive, like an inanimate object, when we're
with friends, and that's not at all the case. On the
contrary, you are aware of everything and you
follow everything that's said and done, but you
have an extraordinary instinct for moderation
and you control perfectly the amount of your
participation in a group of adults.

It's strange that since you were relatively
young you've always preferred to be with
grown-ups. When someone has said at a celebra-
tion or a party: "grown-ups here, the children will
eat at the other table, or in the garden", whoever
was in charge assumed that because of your size,
and also because you're what you are, you would
go with the little ones or with the older children.
Sometimes you did, when it was a party for boys
and girls, but if you had the choice you chose to
be with adults.

Experts talk in terms of the mental age of
people like you, and I must say that I cannot
agree with them. What is your mental age now?
There must be some kind of test which will say
six or eight or ten or whatever, but that is a fallacy
disguised as figures. You can't do sums that a
child of seven could do, but you have an idea of
human behaviour, of social situations, of the

value of what others say, that a child does not have. You don't seem to me to have a childish mind, and I'm sure that to confuse an intellectual coefficient with an authentic mental age is a nonsense. You are seriously incapacitated for learning many things which constitute a traditional school education, but the mind is something different, and your mind functions so correctly in certain aspects – aspects which I value a great deal from a human point of view – that for me it is as adult as your body.

So it is becoming increasingly hard for me to accept the expression "mentally defective" in cases like yours. It is also incorrect to say "psychologically defective", but we'll talk about that another day. If the mind is the cognitive faculty, as the dictionary puts it, the power of understanding, yours is defective in one area; but you are capable of comprehending acts, attitudes, situations with a fine perception that doesn't seem to me in the least childish but mature, and also you interpret them, or react to them, in a rational way.

But I'll leave it at that for the moment, because I'm not writing these pages to set myself up as an expert, or to deny that it is useful – although I don't think it is exact – to continue talking in terms of "mentally defectives"; no, I prefer to talk about you, about how you have come to

have so many friends and how you feel more at
home when you are with adult people.

You've spent hours and hours listening to us
talking, and sometimes I look at you out of the
corner of my eye, and I don't know how it
happens but you are aware of this and give me a
look of complicity which only we understand.
Because you are observant, and you don't fail to
notice when someone is talking in an impas-
sioned or angry fashion, and you look at me in a
way that means "don't you believe it!", with the
irony which is so characteristic of you.

Like me, you are a night-bird. If we're out to
dinner at a friend's house and the talk goes on
until two or three in the morning, you're not
sleepy, you don't want to go to bed. That group
of friends we went with on a trip to Switzerland –
you know who I mean – when we had dinner
with them one Saturday at Argentona and stayed
there for the weekend, Juan and Montse
arranged for us all to have dinner at their
mother's house, because that was where we
were sleeping, so you could go to bed at any time
you wanted. But you stayed to the very end, as
always. As long as there are people and talk no
one can make you go to bed.

I don't really know what you get out of your
silent but sustained and almost stubborn participation. Sometimes you make some comment

afterwards which would make me think that you've taken in fully what was said if I didn't know that that isn't possible. Certainly you miss a lot, because when normal adults talk they usually refer to historical facts or experiences of life that you can know nothing about. My awareness of you has made me realize that we incessantly lace our conversation with threads like "it was when Porcioles was mayor" or "the piazzas of Italy are beautiful but hard". Of course all that kind of allusion means nothing to you, but you never seem bored or abstracted, you go on listening as if you needed to, for some reason that I don't know. That's why you can't understand many of my thoughts, but then neither can I understand everything you think. Tit for tat.

If you do this it must be because you need to, and it would be absurd if through a formal convention – "you ought to go to bed, it's very late" – we imposed ourselves upon your desire for background. We've learnt, I think, not to see you in a petrified way, as a child, but as an individual personality rich in mysteries – for us – whose decisions must be respected. It's only when we think of your defect that we find it illogical that you endure so long and with such contentment a party of adults. But if instead of thinking of what you lack we make the effort to accept that you act in accordance with what you have – and that we know far less about that than about your deficiencies – when you take some decision that surprises us we have to admit that it is an absolutely logical one for you. It is this logic that matters most and that must prevail.

Many of the things we've tried to teach you by means of schools and programmed methods you haven't learnt, but you have equipped yourself with unusual but useful material without our being able to explain how. Is it perhaps because you have a strong desire to absorb everything around you? Is it perhaps because through concentrating so unwearyingly on adults you know that among all the dark clouds you see go by you sometimes glimpse the light of a tiny star, and you can make it yours for ever?

There's a fashionable phrase you've sometimes used yourself, Olga: "That's your problem." If I were a researcher it could be my problem to understand – and I don't really want to – why you so much like being with grown-up people and listening to them, and to understand many other things that I find astonishing. But as I'm only your father, it doesn't matter.

What really does matter, dear Olga, is that you have your solutions, and all we have to do is give you freedom to find them.

5 YOUR FEELINGS

Dear Olga

If I were to talk to you about your psychological condition, you wouldn't understand at all and you'd give me one of those ironic looks which are so typical of you, as though to say "what nonsense are you talking now?" I don't know how the word "psychological" would come out if you said it aloud. With time, you've learnt to speak very acceptably, but there are still words that bog you down. "Clinic", for example. You know you say it wrong, but more especially you know you say it in a funny way which people find amusing: it sounds, more or less, like "clicla" and some-

times sets the whole family roaring with laughter
– and you join in – exaggerating it, and drawing it
out, "cliclicla".

I said in my last letter that I don't agree with
the usual classification of physically defective
and psychologically defective. There's no reason
why those we call subnormal are necessarily
defective psychologically. I don't believe that
you are, and as I don't think of you as a unique
case and believe that your fellow-sufferers, or
many of them, have the same characteristics as
you, the systematic use of the phrase "psychologically defective" seems to me barbaric.

"Psychological" comes from "psyche", which
the dictionary defines as "a term used especially
by psychologists and modern psychoanalysts
instead of 'soul' or 'spirit', referring to the
organized totality of the conscious and
unconscious processes and the intentional
activity of man".

No one will deny that you have plenty of soul
or spirit, or a "psyche" that is as healthy as mine,
or more so, and that your "intentional activity" is
correct. So perhaps they have wanted to include
too many things in the concept "psychological".
You've never needed a psychologist or a psychia-
trist to set right any disturbance in your
"psyche". Your life-world may be more limited
than that of other people, but psychologically

you are perfectly balanced. You are self-aware, you have good relationships with other people, you are extraordinarily good and generous, and you feel happy and say so. Therefore I couldn't include you among the psychologically defective.

There is, on the other hand, evidence that you belong in the class of the intellectually defective, which is a different matter.

There are people who are not intellectually defective, on the contrary, they have a high IQ, but they are psychologically defective in the sense that their "spirit", their "psychological processes" or their "intentional activity" is not of the quality considered as correct. There are people who are mentally very gifted but who are psychologically impaired or sick. Their relatives, their friends, their colleagues at work and, in short, society suffer the consequences. It is these who have to seek the help of psychotherapists – not that of special teachers.

To put it more simply: there are people whose intellectual capacity – I dare not say intelligence, which can mean something else – has developed correctly but whose psychological condition is deformed. There are people, like you, who suffer from intellectual deficiency, and so need special teaching, but whose psychological development has been correct.

I realize that I'm thinking about feelings, but I have to think about your feelings when I'm thinking about you, don't I, Olga?

I like to talk about your goodness, because you aren't exactly an "innocent" in the sense of one who does not know, who is unaware. You know what is bad and that evil exists, and you denounce it indignantly when someone tells you of it or you see it on the television. Your goodness is not a limitation, but a moral decision that you've made and that has grown stronger over the years simultaneously with the development of your conscience.

I've never seen you commit even the smallest bad action.

In the area of principles you have clear ideas, which you can formulate when you think it appropriate. "There must be peace. Between people and in the whole world." "People ought to love one another." "People who aren't good aren't people." When I hear you say these things – so seriously, with so much conviction – it impresses me deeply, Olga, because they are not phrases that you've learnt and are simply repeating, but they show me that you *see* these ideas and are committed to them.

Because you put these principles systematic-ally into practise. Your goodness can be expressed with a word which is hard to swallow–

"sacrifice"; but as you never say it and so avoid the danger of dramatization, I can use it now, although I can express it more exactly. It's not that you sacrifice yourself but that above all else you think about other people's comfort. This is your goodness.

"Let's go and see grandad, he'd like that." Sometimes you use words to express what you feel, but often your goodness is tactfully silent and shows itself in actions, in facts, so it can deceive no one. If I go into a room where you and your mother are watching television and you understand that I am going to stay there for a while, your reaction is not an automatic polite gesture which you've learnt and means nothing: you get up (and that isn't easy with your leg "which is a nuisance", as you say) and you fetch another chair for me, and you move yours away a little so that I get a better view.

If you are watching cartoons, or one of the films you like because they're about a family, and you change channels because there are advertisements or to see what else is on, and you find that there's football or tennis on another channel, you come and tell me at once because you know I'll enjoy it, and other people enjoying themselves is more important to you than "your" film.

This altruism comes absolutely naturally to

you. I don't think we've ever tried to train you against egoism.

Is it because you can't be very useful – or not useful in many ways – that you make up for it by doing as much as you possibly can in anything that depends on you? Probably, but that means you believe that the important thing is to serve, to help, to think of other people all the time. You never miss an opportunity of doing your daily good deed. And of course we don't reward you, we don't treat you as though you were a little child: it would sicken us to see you treated like an amusing little dog at the circus which knows that if it does well it will be given a lump of sugar. We just say thank you, as we do to your brother and sister. We aren't what you might call formal or ceremonious at home.

If you act with goodness it isn't that you do it to win praise or so that we make a fuss of you. We take as much notice of you as we need to; no more, no less.

The simple fact is that you are naturally good-natured, but you know how to mobilize this to do the good within your reach.

So, when we are in your presence how can the rest of us shout at each other or hurt each other? I think that much of the peace and consideration we enjoy at home we owe to you, Olga.

You may be intellectually deficient, but you

are a good example of psychological efficiency, and your feelings act as a regulator of our feelings.

Now you certainly won't understand why I am saying "thank you".

6 LIKING TO DO THINGS

Dear Olga

The first time we went out with you into the street it was a rather strange experience for us, you know (but of course you don't know, luckily), because inevitably people stared at you. Especially because of that "blessed leg" – yes, you're right, Olga, the one which is a bit shorter and makes you limp.

But now it definitely doesn't matter.

When you were a child, when you were younger and you weren't physically very different from other little girls of your age, we often felt uncomfortable as we walked along with you, because people look, and when they see a face, an expression, something not quite ordinary, they stare. It's a very natural instinct, and we realized that and tried to walk on as though there was nothing wrong, and to blot out the unpleasant feeling.

It's a discomfort that can only be cured by repetition.

So I can imagine the tragedy of parents who've never dared take their children out of doors – for years and years there have been handicapped people of all sorts who were made "invisible" – and could never bear the idea of exposing themselves and their children to public curiosity. By hiding their child away they were hiding their insecurity, their fear. It is understandable, because then society was more cruel and unjust because people knew less about it.

It's the same with speaking in public and many other things. The first time your heart thumps, your hands sweat, your legs tremble, but you make up your mind not to be beaten, to get through the rough patch, and you try it again, and each time you mind it less and you end up speaking fairly calmly.

So we decided, in effect, to get through the rough patch because we knew that if we didn't we would lose a mark, but the one who would lose most would be you. Hiding you would mean making you even more "abnormal".

Gradually we must have got used to it, because I suppose people went on staring, but it didn't bother us. Sometimes, I must confess, I used to get annoyed when there was a particularly blatant case – those women who turn round and stop as you go by, and you can see them still standing rooted to the spot, looking after us curiously as we slowly move on; but with equal sincerity I can say that what annoys me is not so much being watched as the fact that such insensitive, such impertinent people exist. Such discourteous people, I mean. If I have learned to be looked at, they ought to have learned to look, because they have plenty of opportunity.

We went to the park to play with other children, didn't we, Olga. I remember the first time you wanted to go down the slide with the others, and in the middle of the others; and we lifted you up on to the swing and gave you a push – just a little one – and away you go . . .

Your mother has had more occasions than me to show her courage. She used to take you to the little square opposite our house and she made friends with other mothers who took their children there. She went with you on buses and on the underground, to the hairdresser and to the dentist. And we went to the beach too – not often, because, I'm sorry, I don't like it – and we dipped you in the sea and we walked up and down over the sand together because it was good for your feet.

I've talked about restaurants before, haven't I? We go there on Saturdays and Sundays because "if it's a holiday, my mother (or my mummy or mamma or mamaruca or whatever you feel like calling her) shouldn't have to get dinner, it's a holiday for her too, see?" Yes, I see. You eat a lot, sometimes I think too much – I don't know where you find room for it inside – but you think it's your duty to eat it all up, although we've told you to eat as you want. You can't deny that you're rather stubborn, even if it is a moral stubbornness. Sometimes you agree, "yes, like a mule". As long as you don't have to chew too hard all is well, you like everything. You were surprised the first time the waiter in a restaurant asked you what you wanted, talking to you like a grown-up person. And you made a very funny face when Carlo who owns the pizzeria called you "Signorinella". When he went away from our table you put your hand half over your mouth so he wouldn't hear you, and tried not to laugh, and you looked more like a kitten than ever as you repeated, in surprise, "Signorinella . . .!"

You've been on excursions and journeys, and

what you remember best is your stay in London with us and your brother and sister. What a lot of walking we did, didn't we? You often had to sit down somewhere – I can still see you taking advantage of a stone bench in a shop in Carnaby Street – because you were tired, but you'd rather have died than have said so. Stubborn, as I said. We saw a lot of things, didn't we? And now when Big Ben comes up on the television, you jump up at once and say, ''That's London!'' And sometimes it doesn't have to be Big Ben, something about a street or a scene makes you say it. You have a good visual memory.

When Josep, your brother, or Gemma, your sister, have taken you on a picnic or to the cinema, how you've enjoyed it! You say, ''I like doing things''.

I understand that well, because we are very alike.

Shall I tell you something, Olga? When we do things together now, when we walk along the street or visit someone or eat in a restaurant, I almost never think of us as a special family.

Nor when I look at you. I've certainly learnt to look at you as you want to be looked at.

7 TO EACH HIS OWN LIFE

Dear Olga

We learnt not to be ashamed of you, which was surely also à way of not feeling ashamed of ourselves, but you've also taught me to see a bit further than just you and me. You've taught me to not be ashamed of other people, or at least to try not to be.

In other words, you've made me think about people and how each individual one of us is what we are.

Is it normal for everyone to have a model of how they think people ought to be? I suppose so, and our model is, obviously, formed on the basis of what we ourselves are or think we are. Other people should adjust to our criteria or, perhaps, adapt themselves to our characteristics – our tastes, ideas, social level – in order to relate more easily to us.

I must make this mistake too, but I shouldn't have realized that it was a mistake – I said that it was normal – if life had not led me to relate to you, Olga. Because you're not a model one could offer as one to be imitated, and at the same time you are a part of my reality, and not a rejected one or one I should be ashamed of, as I said, but a loved and integral part of my consciousness and my sensitivity. This helps a little to lessen my instinctive contempt for those who don't achieve my optimum characteristics.

How can I expect of everyone what I cannot expect of myself? Do people have to be like me to be worth anything?

Years ago I wrote a collection of songs for children, and you learnt a few of them by listening to the records.

On one of them there were songs for the fat boy, the skinny boy, the tall boy, the short girl – do you remember?

> A shorty, a shorty,
> I am a shorty;
> On top of a table
> I look quite high . . .

> But it's not so bad
> To be not very tall,
> For if I tumble down
> I've not so far to fall.

The little short girl was tired of people calling her "midget", and they made fun of the tall one too – "mind out, duck your head, there's a plane coming over" – but they couldn't deny that there were advantages too. The thin one was so very skinny that, "So as not to get wet, when it rains I lie/Underneath a washing line, and there keep dry."

And his school friends have to agree:

> When there's far too many of us
> And we're all squeezed up at table
> We wish we were more like you
> For you don't take up too much room
> And you make yourself quite small.

What a good model we have for the fat one! But:

> Playing football in the playground
> Fatty's side always will win:
> He puts himself in the goalmouth
> No shot can ever get in.
> Here's one thing about Fatty
> That we like him for,
> He never ever loses
> His good temper.

I don't know whether you understand it all, Olga, but I like to remember you singing it cheerfully, and how the whole lot of us produced more than the usual family racket when we sang the one about:

> We're like this, we're like that,
> Tall and short and fat and thin ones.
> We're like this, we're like that,
> Each of us in his own way,
> We'll all get on together.

Each of us in his own way – yes, each with his own life which, as the old bus tickets used to say, is "personal and non-transferable".

Looking at you, I've discovered that differences must be respected. Not only the differences of those who are near to me – which can be accepted through love – but the differences of every individual; and this acceptance can only be achieved – unless one is essentially a saint – as the result of a mental exercise, a calm and even cold analysis of human reality. In the same way that a botanist recognizes and accepts the enormous diversity of the plant world and it never occurs to him to hold up one of them as a model to be imitated, we adults must observe our contemporaries without prejudices which disqualify them on account of what they themselves are and we are not, or do not suppose ourselves to be.

Is there something wrong about fennel because it is not a rose?

If rose-bushes had an egocentric view of the world they would think so.

Unless, perhaps, a little bit of fennel grew from a side-shoot of the rose-bush, and the rose-bush felt it belonged to it.

Although there are thousands of girls like you, Olga, statistics say that you are a minority. The reality is that we are all a minority, and I'm not talking about a select minority, an elite which is identified with superiority. Each individual is a minor existence in the whole species, and what happens is that our sensibility is a magnifying mirror turned inside out so that we see ourselves larger.

It's easy to accept that you are a minority because your particular defect can be analyzed objectively. But your existence has enabled me to take a step further forward, to think a little beyond ourselves and to understand that we are all single entities in comparison with the rest, and that in relation to them we always have a defect, just as they have one for us.

The difference is, Olga, that your defect can be diagnosed scientifically and no one can deny it, and the defects of people like me are debatable, they are part of the market of values which each individual fixes in his own way. So we set up an emotional coefficient, an aesthetic coefficient, a coefficient of cultural interests, a coefficient of social habits, which lead us to look down on those who don't measure up to them (and sometimes to criticize those who go beyond them).

You, Olga, have inoculated me against feeling contempt for the defects of others, and if I am so little intelligent that I can't avoid it, at least I am aware of it. And you've helped me, too, to live with my own defects without being obsessed with them, with a naturalness which – I don't know what moralists will say – seems to me very healthy.

8 WHAT IS PROGRESS?

Dear Olga

Sometimes I've felt a rather uncomfortable doubt: is there something more I could have done for you?

I don't mean about my emotional attitude, I'm quite easy about that. My doubt is whether I've provided you with all the practical possibilities for education and training.

Have I been negligent?

Am I sure that you wouldn't have been able to acquire other knowledge and techniques that you are not mistress of now?

I'm not sure that I've worried enough about

these things, but I must confess that it only occurs to me from time to time, it's a fleeting shadow that passes through my head when someone tells me how his subnormal daughter or son has learnt to type, or can do some form of handiwork better than you.

Perhaps you too might have taken a further step forward; but my scruples soon evaporate. Perhaps it's so as not to distress myself, perhaps because what I think is true: that in your personal case this possibility has or would have only a relative importance. I don't believe that in practice, for a hypothetical tomorrow, this little gain in ability would be really useful to you and would change your situation. It would be another matter if the consciousness of your limitation made you feel frustrated or embittered: then it would be unpardonable to have denied you the opportunity to better yourself.

It's also true that early stimulation methods were not known in Spain when we might have tried them with you. When you were little we were very uninformed, and it was only a few years ago that new educational possibilities were explored. Parents who face the problem today will be well advised to get as much information as they can.

But, dear Olga, there are other things. I remember the doctors telling us that once you had reached puberty – approximately – you wouldn't be capable of further progress. In one area, which is very important for me and for you too, they were wrong.

Because the idea that "everything that has not been learnt by a certain age should be considered unattainable" may be true, but only in a very scholastic sense, of intellectual learning. The fact is that you, as a person, have not come to a halt. As a person you've continued to grow and to develop.

And it was precisely once you had left adolescence behind you that this progress was more obvious to us. I believe that, intellectual coefficient apart, your development is very like that of normal people when they become adults. You've become more aware of what we could call the reality of life, more capable of observing concrete facts, actions and personalities and of drawing entirely rational conclusions from them: your mental associations are richer, your language is more precise and more varied than it was ten years ago; your self-control is more secure and you take decisions more freely and ones that are more your own.

I once wrote an article about people like you which had this title: "The children who will always be children". My intention was good, and perhaps it was useful, but the years have passed and you have shown me that the title was a mistake. You were a child but you are one no longer. Now I have an adult relationship with you that I couldn't have before. When we go out in the car, whenever it happens that you and I are alone together, it never occurs to me that I am with a "child" but I behave, without thinking, as I would with any grown-up person.

I'll go further, Olga, and say that when we're together at home or anywhere else I'm hardly ever aware that you have Down's Syndrome, and this is surely because we have grown used to relating to each other on the basis of what we have in common, of what we can share naturally and fully.

In the light of this fundamental progress I try not to give too much importance to the possible short-fall in what we might call technico-manual training.

You can't deny that you're rather lazy about that sort of thing. Sometimes at home we've asked you to show us how you make that woven material you work on at Boscana, but you've always said no. Probably because you find it taxing, and while you do it there as a matter of discipline, at home you feel free from that kind of obligation. I called you lazy, and that was unfair, because you're never lazy when it's a matter of helping to lay the table, tidying the newspapers,

sweeping, drying up knives and forks and plates
. . . Perhaps the truth is that you're always ready
to do something which is your job at a set place
and time, and you're lazy when you don't feel
obliged to do anything.

I think I understand you, because I'm like
you. I'm not one of those people who have
always to be doing something, who always have
to be productive, who justify their existence by
continuous action. Time to be idle seems to me a
very human time, and so I respect yours. I've
never been able to see you as a machine that
could be made perfect, to whom techniques and
requirements of profitability could be applied,
but as a living human being with inner needs
which others cannot understand (and it is true of
all of us) but which we have to admit.

I, too, have very little manual dexterity, and
I've still less desire to make use of it. I'm not
surprised that in addition to your own particular
difficulty you've inherited my clumsiness, and
for all these reasons I tend to forgive you
whenever you are reluctant to make that kind of
effort.

Could you have achieved better results, then,
in certain other skills? I'm sure you could. So
could I, so could your brother and sister. So
could everyone.

We all fall short of the level which is within

our reach. Sometimes the reason is that we never came across the history teacher – for example – who could arouse our interest in the subject. Or the manager who could stimulate us to accept new responsibilities at work. Or extremely unfavourable family or social or financial circumstances.

Sometimes the reason for not having made more progress is within ourselves.

But, Olga, we don't yet really know what progress is.

I do know, though, that progress is not a single road, an obligatory route for everyone, although our society may believe that it is.

Your special condition gives you the freedom not to submit to the tyranny of a progress which is identified with efficiency and competitiveness. You have gone forward, in your way, in the way of the line by Victor Hugo:

Avançons.

Le progrès, c'est un besoin d'azur.

There is a blue in your life, dear Olga, which grows clearer and deeper, which the most expert hands cannot create.

9 WHAT WE HAVE IN COMMON

Dear Olga

I was telling you that you and I, each in our own way, have little manual dexterity, and that when you feel like being lazy I can sympathize with you.

I think that we have a lot of things in common, and that is a further proof that there is no such thing as a stereotyped subnormal person, nor is there any uniform pattern for a Down's Syndrome person.

Like any other child, a Down's person constructs his or her character with the mysterious but certain materials of genetic inheritance and the no less subtle but unquestionable materials provided by his or her environment. The child born with Down's Syndrome isn't a finished product but a human being who can change and develop through the influences he or she receives.

You and each one of your fellows differ by reason of the sum of the two kinds of characteristics, the innate and the acquired.

What is there in your intellectual equipment that is related to mine, apart from a distaste for pottering about or for spending time on manual work?

To make up for it, a remarkable capacity for attentiveness, perhaps favoured by very acute hearing. We both have to wear glasses, and mind it much more than anyone supposes, in my case because of age and in yours because of your condition. Sometimes I think that the same thing happens with you as with me, that you're able to follow two different conversations at the same time, but in any case your hearing is out of all proportion to your other faculties. At home your "ears" are important, and you often warn us of sounds – the lift, a pan boiling over in the kitchen – which no one else has noticed. We've learnt that we can't make any kind of *sotto voce* comment in your presence. You hear it, and I sometimes think that you hear it partly because you can partly guess what it is – it happens to me sometimes too. We have a certain ability, you and I, for interpreting that has nothing to do with intelligence, or at least with pure intelligence, if such a thing exists. I think that it's nothing but a strange kind of agility, a swiftness of perception that enables us to associate and piece together fragmentary clues. In my case, because of my temperament and because of the sort of work I do, it is perhaps not surprising that I should have developed this aptitude; but that you should have the same gift, relatively speaking, for this attentiveness never ceases to surprise me.

Is your irritation in the face of group disloyalty hereditary too? I'll explain what I mean. I've a feeling, which must be an unhealthy one, that in a social situation everyone should behave in the way appropriate to him or her. For example, when in a gathering where it has been decided to listen to some music someone starts a conversation with the person sitting beside him, or when someone suddenly puts on a record during a conversation that is interesting and going well. Often at a concert I find it wrong when one of the musicians who has a few bars rest glances round or looks uninterested – as if for those few moments he wasn't part of the orchestra – instead of showing solidarity with his companions who are still playing.

I've given this example, Olga, because I

remember sometimes at Christmas or end-of-term festivities at Boscana how you've reacted if one of the girls stopped taking part in the song you were singing and started to chatter to the girl next to her, or waved to her parents at the back of the hall. Your look of indignation was very expressive, you couldn't help it, and when you thought the audience couldn't see you, you even rebuked her (but if it would have interrupted the continuity of the performance, you swallowed your recriminations so as not to commit the same fault).

We have to acknowledge, dear Olga, that you and I have another thing in common: we have a rather exaggerated idea of the respect due towards an attitude which seems to us to be called for. The truth is that we give too much importance to those "liberties" people take which most people find normal. In my case this results in my being thought disagreeable, because people know about this nonconformity of mine and "it's not as important as all that". In your case, however, your need for collective obligation is rather agreeable to anyone who is aware of it, and for me it is both very pleasing and also very impressive to see myself portrayed in your attitude. Portrayed in a positive way: the wish to respect one rule for all; and in a negative way: the difficulty of tolerating exceptions.

We share another curious attribute: the ability to improvise words to music we know. Do I do it at home from time to time? I suppose so, and you've probably heard your mother do it too, because if not it would be hard to imagine why you should do such a thing. But it's undeniable that you have a natural facility for it, like me, and that you manage extremely well to make the phrase you improvise fit into the musical phrase. One day when I was taking you to school you started singing to the music of *L'Estaca* – "If you will stretch him out full length" – inventing the words "it will be Christmas, Christmas, soon,/ and holidays for Olga".

Apparently many Down's children appreciate music, but this is something different, an instinct for invention and adaptation – more or less well – to the rhythm. Sometimes I've started the exercise and encouraged you to carry on, and you've always added words to my words, following the cadence of the music and even making the necessary vocal adjustments – spreading a syllable over two notes, for example – so as to stay faithful to the melody as far as you could. For some people that must be harder than to make up a proper text. For you and me it's much easier.

Another common trait: visual memory.

Careful now! I don't mean that you have an extraordinary visual memory, because normal children certainly have as much as you, or more. Certainly? Yes, although sometimes I've thought that you compensate for the poverty of your resources in other channels of perception by increasing your visual intake (just as blind people are said to develop a more than normally acute sense of hearing). But if we go past a house you've only seen once when we went to visit someone there, your ability to identify it again visually surprises us. But this is in comparison with your other "instruments of perception". Your brother and sister, when they were little, already had more visual memory than you have now, but I didn't give it much thought because it wasn't exceptional in them.

What do I mean by all this, dear Olga? That I too have a visual rather than an historical memory? Yes, but above all I'm telling you that it moves me to feel that I am your father and that I share with you so many abilities, and so many ineptitudes.

10 MY SECRETARY

Dear Olga

I can't put myself inside your brain and know what you're thinking when I see you gazing out of the window or thumbing through the pages of a magazine you don't understand.

Because I'm sure that like everyone else you're always thinking, but I don't know if your mechanism for reflection is different from ours, or the same even though perhaps – perhaps – poorer. And when I say poorer I feel that I'm on unsure ground, because I don't know if I mean technically poorer – in speed, precision in the process of forming ideas – or poor in content, in results.

On the other hand, are some thoughts worth more than others?

In the minute during which I've elaborated a series of ideas on the football match I'm watching you may have had only one thought: "Now my father is happy." (Sometimes you say to me "there's football – or tennis – today, you're happy, aren't you?".) I have the impression that I think more, but the question is still an open one: what thoughts are more worth thinking? There are people who are incapable of thinking in the course of a day: "I feel alive, I love you, how peaceful it is at the moment, what a nice noise those bells make!"

What do you think about?

I mean, what are you thinking about when you don't say anything? Because when you tell me I know, and I like to know what you are thinking, but when I come to consider it I realize that you're not talkative, that you have many periods of silence – and instead you listen very attentively – and that when you speak it is to say something very concrete. You never say any-thing pointless, you never speak in vain. You don't tell us about the unimportant things at school, but facts – summarized – which may interest us. You don't talk about yourself. You haven't the nervous habit of repeating conven-tional phrases with inappropriate insistence, which happens in some cases. It's as if you kept your limited repertory of self-expression well under control, as if you had the intelligence to make correct use of your reduced allocation of intelligence.

Or as if you had the instinct to do it, which comes to the same thing.

So you're never boring, you never interrupt a conversation, and none of our friends has ever considered you an intrusion.

Sometimes I'd like it if you joined in more when we're with friends, just to know what you're thinking. Your notable tact is a great quality, and I'm grateful to you for it because it has been and is very convenient for us, and it has helped us to make your social life a normal one. But now I shall make a resolution: the next time you are present during a conversation among my friends – the sort of conversation that goes on for a long time and touches on many different sub-jects – at a certain moment I shall ask you what you think about what we're discussing.

Perhaps you won't be able to explain, but you will certainly have been thinking something. I'm sure that it will be not at all nonsense, though it will certainly be very elementary. But as you listen and follow the conversation – follow it in your own way – you must surely be having ideas. If it's practice you lack, then I must encourage you more often to express your impressions of what you are experiencing.

I know, Olga, that your world is narrower than mine. I don't mean in feelings or emotions – who can compare, qualitatively, those of two individuals? – but the cultural world of enquiry, observation, interests.

Your circle of interests is a small one (but they are very intense interests, surely because they are few in number). Questions of politics, ecology, labour, any kind of championship, fashion and clothes, discotheques, youth problems, public security, holidays, money – hardly touch you. None of that forms part of your world, or you take it all as it comes.

You are only concerned about a few things, and to those you give thought.

In this sense, Olga, I've exploited you, because you act as my secretary.

How I like to call you my secretary, don't I!

I know that it's a bit of an exaggeration, and if anyone knew that I've called you my secretary they'd think that I'm rather silly. You have none of the qualifications expected even of a very low-grade normal secretary, and the truth is that you couldn't do any practical task for me that would free me from having to do it myself.

But sometimes I trust you more than anyone else, when it's a matter of remembering small things. It's as though you were my "emergency diary".

For example: "Olga, remind me when we go out that I've got to take this parcel." Or: "Before I drop you off at school I must take this article to the office."

You never fail. Often I don't forget either, but more than once I've been saved trouble thanks to you. Someone phoned just as I was going out, or I've wanted to make sure I had enough tobacco on me, or something else unforeseen has put it out of my mind – and just as I reached the landing I'd hear your voice: "What about the parcel?"

And another time, seeing which way the car was going, you've warned me "What about that article?"

Yes, Olga, you were on the alert.

Then you're happy, you feel useful, and it's nice when you say, "If it hadn't been for me . . .", or you make that expressive little grimace which means, "My poor father, he's hopeless!"

Yes, for these things I rely more on you than on your brother or sister, and the reason is obvious: they – like your mother, like me – are involved in many things, they have their own concerns, their own headaches, and my request is added to their agenda as an extra burden, and it's easy for it to get obliterated by some more personal or immediate interest. Your world, as I said, is narrower. My request enters on its own and becomes an important piece of news for you. For a time you are "the person who has to remind me of something". And usually you do it, and you do it very well because you don't become obsessed with it and remind me over and over again, but you keep it to yourself, and confine yourself to watching me and only save me from the oversight when I'm on the point of committing it.

At home, if we don't want to overlook something the solution is simple: "We'll tell Olga."

Your world is narrow, but there's always room in it for other people.

11 I DON'T WANT TO KNOW "WHY?"

Dear Olga

You are as you are from a cause that you'll never understand: a genetic change characterized by the presence of an extra chromosome. Having more than necessary makes you less than normal.

·This superfluous chromosome has prevented you from developing correctly, and here is an apparent paradox: you were born defective because of an excess. But the phenomenon is not as rare as it seems, in the sense that the same contradiction is produced in other aspects of the human personality: an excess of sensitivity, for example, can become pathological; and no one would deny that affection is a good thing, but an excess of protective affection in infancy can produce an abnormality.

Excess is often dangerous, and not only an unfavourable excess such as a very restricting family poverty, but also an excess that could be considered favourable, such as a superabundance of money or of facilities. Growing up in an over-favourable situation constitutes no guarantee of success.

We don't know how the change which produces Trisomy 21, which is the excess chromosome you have, takes place, and to tell the truth I consider my ignorance on this point of little or no importance. (The fact that I want experts to investigate it, and to find out whether there is any way of avoiding or correcting this error of nature, is another matter.) It doesn't worry me now, and it never has worried me. Your birth landed us with a lot of problems, but no question-mark.

What mattered was the fact, and the fact was there and irreversible, and we had to make it part of our future.

A variety of causes can produce subnormalities, and some occur after birth. Sometimes it's possible to find an explanation for them and even, in some cases, the explanation is human negligence.

No one is to blame for your problem, Olga, and on this point the parents of children like you have to put out of their minds from the very start any suspicion of doubt or anxiety. This doesn't always happen, unfortunately. I know some very sad cases of a father or mother who has sought to extricate themselves from the reality that was burdening them with accusations or suspicion against the other.

You and the others like you, Olga, do something that is really very hard: you put adults to the test, and sometimes it is evident that the adults are not very adult. They react with a kind of obstinacy, with that immaturity that leads us to reject some mishap, some failure in our lives, what we call adversity, and when this happens we have to pass on responsibility for it to someone else.

I don't want to know why you were born like this, Olga. If scientists can explain by what mechanism the disruptive chromosome is produced, they should keep the discovery to themselves until they find a way to prevent it in the future. If they know already, and if the causative factor can be found in the father or the mother they should not give us a technical explanation. It frightens me to think of the harm that could be done to some couples by the disclosure of "technical responsibility". A Down's child demands from the parents a great commitment, an obligation of solidarity, an acceptance on equal terms. If now, when we are ignorant of the causes it is still sometimes very difficult to reach the only possible constructive attitude, which is "it's happened to both of us", the possibility of knowing "which one of us – unwittingly! – it comes from" makes the problem potentially terribly destructive: "It's happened to both of us but it's nothing to do with me, it's your affair."

Fortunately you've been our affair for so long, dear Olga, that no verdict that would differentiate between us could affect your mother or myself. But in the case of young parents who've not yet had time to bind themselves in the sort of solidarity I've described, such precision could be disastrous and arouse the pathology of scruples, aggression, guilt complex . . . and confrontation not only between parents but between two families.

It seems to me much healthier both for the child and the parents to accept the statistical mischance. Of every six hundred children born, one is affected by Down's Syndrome. This is a percentage which is more or less constant in all countries, all social classes, all races. We've been unlucky, really. The law of probability allowed us to be confident, but it turned out against us.

It turned out against some of our friends and acquaintances too, and against many unknown people, some of whom have come to me from time to time over the years, to tell me their experiences and to listen to what I could tell them. And what could I tell them? When they went away I've always felt dissatisfied. Perhaps now I would let them read these letters I'm writing for you, Olga, but can anyone say anything really useful to parents who still ask – and it's natural that they should ask, it will be a long time before the question ceases to have any importance – "Why did it happen to *us*?"

I'm afraid they've often found my words, of guidance or of solidarity, too superficial. Perhaps they've even thought that I didn't feel sorry enough about the misfortune that had afflicted them because I didn't show it with the usual signs.

Of course I felt sorry, but it must be an instinct – I don't know if it's a sound one or a wrong one – which prevents me from sentimentalizing on the subject. I said that perhaps they found me too superficial because instead of spending time in mutual commiseration I've gone straight to the consideration of concrete aspects of the situation they consulted me about, and made practical suggestions – as if it were a matter on which one could think calmly, constructively, and not a matter which may have completely overturned people's way of life.

I must be a bad counsellor, but I'd like to think that in the long run it has been useful to people who have come to me spontaneously – and perhaps gone away disappointed – that they have seen me so little downcast. Because I'm convinced that one of the functions of those of us who have already lived through the problem is to help those who are facing it to "de-obsess" themselves. It is a mistake – for oneself and for the child – to confuse obsession with responsibility. One must keep one's head clear and one's feelings calm in order to organize appropriately a personal and family life that has been touched by Down's Syndrome.

So it is important to reject useless and destructive questions and settle for the statistical explanation. We've been unlucky, that's all. And what do we do when we meet with bad luck in whatever our field of activity may be? We have to see what we can do to make up for it.

And you, dear Olga, are at the same time our bad luck and our compensation.

I'll tell you later what I mean.

12 WHAT DOES "HUMAN LIFE" MEAN?

Dear Olga

You don't know what "subnormal" means, but neither do many intelligent adults. If they knew what lies behind the word "subnormal" they wouldn't use it so unthinkingly.

Because they turn it into an insult, like "dimwit" or "half-wit". What a bad joke, isn't it Olga, to insult someone by telling them that their intelligence is below normal, as if to have a below-average intelligence were a crime, a sin, a vice, a fault? It's like insulting someone by saying that they were blind from birth, or deaf, or disabled.

If they wouldn't dare reprimand a subnormal person by shouting "dimwit", why do they not hesitate to shout it at anyone? It's not maliciousness, I know, it's thoughtlessness, it's lack of sensitivity. After all, they use the expression to insult people who actually know what mentally defective people are really like, and so I'm driven to think that it's a word with a conventional value which in a social context goes beyond its actual meaning. The same sort of thing happens with "bastard" used as an insult to someone who does something we disapprove of, and as such we often hear it on the lips of progressive and "enlightened" people who don't realize that they are contributing to the idea that to be born to an unmarried mother is reprehensible.

So "subnormal!" used as an insult causes great distress to those of us who are sensitive to the condition of such people, but we can realize that not everyone has stopped to think about it.

What I find hardest to understand, dear Olga, is that some people take their thoughtlessness and bad manners – I won't say malice, because there is none – to the point of insulting people like you in a basic and public way. It means they know nothing about you.

Only three years ago a woman who held an important position made a statement to the press about abortion. She said: "The approved withdrawal of penalties is a minimum concession. If I myself had found myself pregnant at the age of fifteen and unmarried, I don't know what I should have done. If I became pregnant now, at the age of forty, I should not have an abortion. However, if I knew that there was a ninety-nine per cent possibility that I would give birth to a subnormal child, then I should, because that would be ridiculous, that is not a human life."

When I read that and I looked at you, dear Olga, I felt a strange heat spreading through me. It was as if someone had tried to say that all the good things we had created between us day by day were false.

I respected that lady, and I still do, she seems to me a very worthy person in many respects. And we all slip up, we all make mistakes from time to time. The danger is that the error may become a permanent judgement, reinforced and formulated like a verdict.

I also respect her freedom to make a decision in a matter of conscience which – in the case of the woman who made the statement – is a complicated and delicate one: she would have an abortion if she knew she had a ninety-nine per cent chance of having a subnormal child. In some cases it is now possible to know. In other cases the chance is ten per cent, twenty per cent, forty per cent. What percentage of risk is acceptable?

But what I can't accept, obviously, is that "it is not a human life".

And it is precisely because of you, Olga, that I cannot accept this dogmatic verdict, because you have helped me understand that what she said about "human life" is a much more subtle and debatable reality than it would seem. Perhaps it is easier to agree on biological "life", but "humanity" is an abstract concept in which many varying interpretations, evaluations, prejudices and so on may enter. Can we call really "human" a life dominated by an obsession with money, or by a rigid egotism, and so on?

Let's leave the subject.

When the lady said that it wasn't a "human life" I suppose she was referring to the subnormal child, but she might have imagined that the parents in such a situation were condemned to an inhuman existence. And I expect that since her words were so unfortunate it was because she hadn't had an opportunity to live with the problem close at hand and that she had formed her opinion through some very negative accounts.

There's no doubt that it's preferable not to have to live with the problem close at hand, but in that case it's advisable to be tactful when the time comes to give an opinion, and especially not to generalize. Because there is as great a diversity among subnormal people – mental defectives, character defectives, etc. – as there is among normal ones. Certainly some types of aggressive, antisocial or autistic subnormality can seriously affect family relationships, as in the case of other sick people: alcoholics, drug-addicts, psychopaths, etc. It is understandable that in a situation of great stress, especially if it becomes chronic, someone may think "this is no sort of life".

Living with these types of subnormal cases may make the life of those around them "inhuman" because there isn't adequate equipment or social service, because society – not the sufferers – is "inhuman". But these inconvenient subnormal people also have a life which, although it isn't as privileged as ours, is equally human.

How many parents and how many teachers, dear Olga, have spoken about you and your companions in a very different way from the lady in the paper! They have spoken from direct experience of the revelatory discovery of the special and profound "humanity" – desires, feelings, pleasures, sorrows – of the "human beings with a difference".

Alongside the tragic cases of co-existence, which must be resolved, are other very different ones. I've never regretted having struggled from your very first day, Olga, for your difficult survival. Intellectual deficiency is one thing; the affection, the good-will to help everyone, the capacity for happiness you possess is another. I am more intelligent than you, but I'm not sure that I am more human. In any case, I know that everything in me that is pure, tender, peaceful, non-egoistical, is largely your work.

To have a subnormal child is not an experience to be desired. But I should be the undesirable one if over the years I had not come to realize that you and I, Olga, have both been enriched by our mutual love and also by our mutual training – yes, I have learnt from you too.

13 YOUR PEACE AND YOUR HEAVEN

Dear Olga

Sometimes when you arrive at our house at Solius, in the middle of the woods, you take a deep breath and you say, "How peaceful!"

You like the different manifestations of peace, one of which is peaceful surroundings. You feel at ease in the silence of nature, stretched out in a deckchair among the trees.

And you like shared peace, peace in company, and we agree on that point too: nature in a "pure" state soon wearies me – the deep forest, the immense, solitary sea – and on the other hand I find it extraordinarily evocative when I see it discreetly accompanied by its counterpart, the human presence: a ploughed field at the edge of an oak wood, a farmhouse in a clearing, a windmill, a boat skirting the coast.

You like it at the weekend when there are people in some of the other houses at Solius. "They are my friends," you say. Yes, they are, and sometimes you ignore the discomfort of your leg to go off on your own to visit them. Among the most friendly people are the monks and the abbot, who treat you with such affection and send you a card on your saint's day.

I was going to say "we all seek peace", Olga, but I'm not so sure. I think some people never do because they don't know it exists, or don't know how to look for it if they do want to find it.

And the truth is that we don't always have to go to the country, to solitude, to find peace, because sometimes people can give it to us. You, for example. To be in contact with you is to live a moment of peace, because anyone who tries having a little conversation with you lives with you for a while, and without realizing it puts out of his head and his heart everything that is an obstacle to communication with your ingenuousness. I know that the word "ingenuous" is often used pejoratively or with a tone of commiseration – "he's so ingenuous" – which is an indication of the prestige that malice, mistrust and the habit of dissimulation have acquired in our society. But when I say ingenuous I'm praising, or perhaps more exactly I'm just defining, one of your positive qualities, Olga. In Roman law the ingenuous person was one who was born free. You were born free of falsity, of ill intention, of possessive ambition.

Anyone who comes across you knows or feels this, and can choose between ignoring you or making contact with you. However brief the period of this contact may be, he has to bring himself to your level of ingenuousness, where aggressive competitiveness makes no sense, and in making the decision to release himself for a little while from the role he has to play in the adult world he will find an interlude of peace.

There is peace in the mountains and in the garden of the monks of Solius, but it is also within you, and you transmit it to others. You are the cobweb-brush that sweeps into our corners where irritation, envy and egoism lie in wait to weave a trap that may hold prisoner our enjoyment of living.

But your love of peace is not defensive, it is not only a concern for your personal comfort. You mind about social peace, about world peace. Your channels of perception are necessarily more limited than mine but you sometimes give me news that you have heard discussed or have listened to on the television, and you explain to me with indignation that there is a war or that there has been some assassination attempt.

One day you said something very amusing: "I don't know why priests talk so much if people don't take any notice!" You like priests – like Father Juan at school – and the monks, because they are affectionate towards you and you hear them talk about love and peace. You'd like everyone to love one another, and you don't understand why they don't. You've not learnt the reasons that explain dislike or hatred, and you've kept your own profound reason. And you are consistent, because you love everyone. I've never found in you any sign of emotional discrimination, and if at times someone who really loves you has treated you with unnecessary harshness you've commented, "He's like that sometimes, I know," and your feelings have never wavered.

You, Olga, are a practising Christian. At school you've received religious teaching – elementary, at your own level – but you've only been able to learn the forms, the formulae. The reality is that you live with a consistent attitude of giving and of tolerance towards others that for me is the basis of Christian spirituality.

You have a conscience that can distinguish categorically between good and evil: good is

love, evil is violence. You've never struck
anyone, I've never seen you make an aggressive
gesture, I've never heard you utter an insulting
or wounding word. And that's not because you
are incapable of it: you have a gift for irony and
for amusing – not destructive – criticism of some
human behaviour; so you are capable of reflec-
ting and reacting. It isn't because of incapacity, as
I said, that you're not violent but because you are
peaceable from choice.

For you, everyone who dies goes to heaven.
Death has already given you sorrow, and you
remember from time to time friends of mine who
had known you ever since you were born, like
Fede or Gloria. Now they are in heaven, you say.
I don't know what heaven is for you. I shall never
tell you that I don't believe in the heaven that I
was taught about, but when you ask me,
"They've gone to heaven, haven't they?" – I
agree with you whole-heartedly, because in
effect they have.

To your heaven. I believe in your heaven,
and, moreover, I believe that there is a place in it
reserved for me. Heaven, dear Olga, is the ulti-
mate gesture of goodness that you send to people
from your heart.

On the other hand, you never talk about hell,
and I think you know nothing about it. It must be
that the monks and the priests and the nuns you

have met have said nothing about it, and I'm grateful to them for that.

I'm very pleased that you never talk about hell and that you often talk about peace. Make no mistake, Olga, peace must exist and hell cannot exist. After so many years with you, I'm well aware of that.

14 A FATHER'S ROLE

Dear Olga

Or perhaps to make my point I should begin "Dear daughter": I have no vocation for parenthood.

A vocation is defined as "a disposition or natural inclination to the exercise of a profession, a skill, etc." and in that great thick book you see me consult sometimes there are two examples given: artistic vocation; vocation for teaching.

I have no vocation for fatherhood nor have I ever had one, at least in the way that I see most men I know possess one, that is, a disposition to act as a father according to the customs prevailing in our society.

There are quite a number of families with children in which the wife addresses her husband as "dad", and the husband calls the wife "mother" or "mum".

That doesn't happen in our house. At home my wife and I always call each other by our names, and we do the same to our children, instead of saying "son" or "daughter". I've always felt that the status of father – like that of writer – was an acquired attribute which couldn't replace or alter the permanent and more fundamental condition of a person.

The fact that I had no vocation for parenthood doesn't mean that I didn't want to act as a father in accordance with my conscience. As it turns out, the view I had, and still have, of my role as a parent – a role that I have to do my best to fulfil but which I don't identify with my status as an "actor" in this life – does not entirely coincide with the views held by other parents I know.

Some people might think that my lack of vocation is explicable precisely by the fact of being the father of a daughter like you. In the sense that people might think it, I'm convinced that they are wrong. I think that your brother Josep, who is married, and your sister Gemma, who is still living at home, would both agree that

I'm right: it's because I'm the sort of person I am, and not because of your existence, that I'm not the usual sort of father.

I'll tell you, Olga, the sort of person I'm not. I'm not a man who studied for a career and who practises it (I don't practise it) or who has inherited or set up a business which constitutes his "work" (which he sometimes confuses with his life) or who has a clearly defined place of work with salary increases, holidays and overtime (I've never had anything resembling that). Perhaps connected with this is the fact that neither am I a man who is happy buying a cine-camera when he has some money to spare, or buying a better car than the one he has (after seven years of owning a SEAT 127 I had another 127 for six years) or redecorating the flat more grandly. I'm not the sort of man who when he's at home has "his" armchair or "his" place at the head of the table or is served first or gets the best part of the joint (not because anybody wants to refuse it to me but because it's obvious that sort of thing isn't important to me). In other words, I've never tended to formalize my existence.

When it came to acting as a parent I accepted it as a possibility of taking part in a process rather than as an obligation to produce a finished product to a given model. Don't think, Olga, that your father is proud of what he's saying. Not at all. I say simply that I realize that I haven't acted, nor do I act, as other parents do, friends of mine whom I deeply respect and can sincerely congratulate.

Perhaps I haven't been a parent by vocation because for many years I've believed that vocations are dangerous when we want others to appreciate our total dedication, our binding commitment. Yes, years ago I understood that the danger into which many parents-by-vocation fall was that they didn't want to bring up children with vocations but children designed according to the parents' vocation. And that changing times – and the media and the children's multiple relationships and new ways of life, etc. – decreased the importance of the designing function of their parents.

I never had the heart, dear Olga, to control the development of your brother and sister. I tried to open up every possibility so that they could find the vocation of realizing themselves in their own time, because, given the rapid evolution of the present generation, in the inheritance that adults are able to pass on there are many actions and many obligations which are outmoded.

I'm not what you could call a child-lover. Is it perhaps exaggerated to say that some people treat their children as "objects" upon which they pour out undeniably real feelings? I've always seen them as adults in embryo, and hence as persons who from the first moment of life are not "mine", whose progressive independence I have to encourage. I believe this is my duty as a parent, and my justification must be that when they're grown-up they continue to be fully "other people" in relation to me.

I'm not against the "family". On the contrary, I grew up in a happy family, with parents of extraordinary goodness, and I deeply love our Christmas gathering – with my eighty-seven-year-old father at the head of the table, and my brothers and sisters and brothers-in-law and sisters-in-law, my children, my nephews and nieces and my grandson. And you, Olga, sit at the other end of the long table, and you see how contented we all are to be together.

But it can't be helped, I've more vocation as a child of a family than as head of a family. I've a greater facility for receiving influences than I have desire to pass them on. I know that whether I want it or not I do have influence – we all do – and I should like to have influenced you, dear Olga, and your brother and sister, in everything that could be useful to you and readily assimilated. But for better or for worse I have no vocation for directing that inevitable general influence towards any specific conditioning.

I've had no vocation as a parent of normal

children nor as the parent of a subnormal daughter. I've never treated you as a child, Olga, but as a defective adult. And who knows if what I told you a little while ago – that I'm the sort of father I am because of my temperament and my ideas and not because I've had you – is only partly true. Who knows if the experience of having you, the great respect I have for your difference, has made me value more highly the independence of each individual, and of your brother and sister, and that as a result I believe that my role as a parent is simply to be at hand, but not to do what must be the normal and perhaps the convenient thing, which I see as an intrusion.

15 ASKING FOR NOTHING

Dear Olga

You can't know that the vast majority of people expect certain things from life or, to express it in a more fashionable way, they have objectives.

What's your aim in life, what do you mean to do, where do you want to get, what do you hope to achieve . . .? These are the things that people ask each other and that many ask themselves. It's a matter of programming, of planning, of having projects . . . Probably it's impossible to live without having some specific intentions.

But you don't have the objectives that normally direct people's thoughts and activities: to marry; to have sexual relations – and this is a subject that for many years has been suppressed in analysing the situation of subnormal people, and which is now being discussed a little; anyway, we've never seen you with any sort of uneasiness in this direction; to have a job that pays (in money, in satisfaction); to have a home; to improve one's social or cultural level; to have children of whom one can feel proud; to save for tomorrow; to make sure of a reasonable pension. You don't hope from life any of these things which are so common.

What you do hope for is much more modest and more immediate, very concrete things: that it won't rain at the weekend so that you can go out, that on the television this evening there'll be the sort of film about families that you like, and not one about war, that we'll go to your party at Boscana, that we'll send you a postcard if we're away on a journey, that your grandmother feels better.

So your horizon of objectives is limited as to what you want to achieve in practical terms, although the range of your grand desires is very ambitious: that we should live for ever, that we should all love one another and be happy . . .

It is the intermediate zone of desires, such as the professional, economic and social ones I've mentioned, that is lacking in you, and these are the ones which usually generate people's normal hopes and often lead to inevitable tensions and frustrations.

But you, dear Olga, only ask for life, and life proportionate to your condition.

Not only are you left on the sidelines of competitiveness, but you also have a very nice trait: you are not at all possessive, and, further-more, you are not a bargainer, a trader. You do what you have to do and ask for nothing in return.

You've made me think about this deep-rooted human tendency to have objectives, the struggle to achieve them, the weapons of obligation and of retribution, of tit-for-tat. It's obvious that this system in human relationships is not only usual but permissible.

But it so happens that I can't adopt this attitude – or this social doctrine – as the sole pattern of my life. And you are the reason for this.

It's easy to understand why: I can't ask you for anything in return.

In return for you being my daughter or me being your father.

In return for taking care of you over the years, and trying to solve your problems.

In return for some petty desire that I've had to

give up for your sake, or in return for a great love.
It doesn't matter.

I can't ask anything of you in return for
anything whatever. And this is the lesson you
have taught me: in life we don't always have the
right to claim retribution for our contribution.

We have to accept that we must do some
things for free. It's a good thing to realize this,
and I thank you for it.

I say "for free" because I deliberately didn't
want to say through "generosity". Generosity
seems too important an idea, and anyway it isn't
applicable in our case. Generosity sounds like a
virtue or at least it supposes a free and merito-
rious giving, whereas I have a duty (or rather,
duties) towards you, and these obligations
include that of doing things "for free", that is,
without asking that they should be repaid.

One of the great problems of emotional
relationships is that they are relationships that
require a certain repayment. It happens between
married couples, between friends, and between
parents and children. Nowadays there are still
many mothers and fathers who persist in the
traditional requirement that children should
show gratitude for everything their parents have
done for them. (A nuance: they don't have to be
grateful at all, but they have to show it.) And
they have to show it not in the way that seems

logical to the child, but in the way the parents require it.

There is always the danger that the understandable desire to be repaid may be converted into moral blackmail. "After all we've done for you . . ." It is obviously intolerable that after all his parents have done for him their son does his hair in a way they don't like. Heavens, what ingratitude! If only it didn't sometimes happen that this leads to tragedies, you and I, Olga, would have a good laugh about it!

There are husbands and wives and friends and parents who always want to be repaid, in one way or another, for what they have done. Children have to repay with good marks at school, or by taking certain subjects, or by going out with girl A instead of girl B, or by giving up an outing with friends because parents want them to go away with them that weekend or for those holidays . . .

As if to have fed and reared a child was an investment which generated a predetermined interest . . .

I think that the sentence should be completed like this: "After all we've done for you – now it's up to you to do what you think best for yourself."

I can't ask anything of you, Olga, in return for what I've done for you, and I've known this for a long time. This realization has led me to keep the same "for free" attitude towards your brother and sister, and this was very fortunate, because compensating for your inability to "repay" me in the way that parents usually claim as a right could have put an excessive burden on them.

You are very limited, they say, and they are right. But at the same time you are an inexhaustible source of ideas. You have broadened my internal horizon, dear Olga, and you have made room there for some actions "for free" – not as many as I would like – and they are those which never oppress one with resentment nor worry one over profitability.

16 NO MORE THAN AN APPROXIMATION

Dear Olga

I'm sorry that it never occurred to me, over all these years, to note down the things you've said which have surprised me.

I remember that long ago there used to be on the television an advertisement for Starlux. I think that one was suddenly shown two cows colliding and simultaneously one heard a typical musical jingle and a voice-over saying, "Starlux double-strength soup."

You were very small, and with the other girls at your school you used to have fun climbing up and going down a slide. Once you were watching some of them do this, and at a certain moment one of the girls started going down before the one before her had got out of the way. And as you watched them collide, you had the acuteness to sing that little jingle: "Starlux double-strength soup"!

You sometimes have quick reactions of this sort, with the kind of humour which amuses me, and what impresses me most is that you don't say these things to anyone, you don't think you are being amusing or want to show off, but they are comments that you make to yourself. Usually you make them quietly, and I'm sure I've missed many of them.

You also have a tendency to invent or alter words, and your mother, who does it too, must have been the influence here. I don't know where she got the little song that goes: "The sea is warmibiris, warmibiris, madam, and it is very nicibiris, nicibiris, to swim . . ." One day she went on to say something to you, I can't remember what, and she began "Listen, Olgabiris . . ." Now you say it yourself from time to time, not for any particular reason but when it seems to you that the atmosphere feels suitably relaxed, or you realize that the conversation has a festive air. For example, if you've made a Christmas card for us, you hide it behind your back and you may say to us, "Now you'll see what Olgabiris has brought for you . . ."

It's as if you make up for your limited means of expression with a strange perceptiveness which ensures that what you say always fits the situation. There must be some explanation because on the one hand you don't know many of the words which are basic to culture and on the other hand you have a certain verbal curiosity. It's as if in your brain you are trying to develop a degree of inventiveness so as to overcome by an instinct the barrier that deprives you of knowledge.

Not all the phrases you've invented and that I wish I'd recorded are amusing, Olga, like the Starlux one. There's another kind, and I shall always remember what you said when you made your first communion. You'd already had that serious infection which destroyed your hip-joint. How difficult it had been for you to learn to walk! We were afraid that in your condition you would never manage to do it again, but you've always been incredibly strong-willed. With will-power and patience, helping yourself along with chairs, with sticks, somehow or other, little by little, you began to conquer. The day of your first communion you walked, hobbling, with a stick. We were in anguish as we watched you move along like that. When the ceremony was over you came towards us and said, with deep and happy conviction, "How lucky I am to be able to walk again!"

I admire your will to be happy, Olga, to see always the favourable aspects of reality. Once you had grown up and were aware of your difficulties of movement, when sometimes you've referred to them it has been with a touch of ironic detachment, making tranquil fun of yourself a little: "This Olgabiris is a cockatoo." It seems as though nothing can make you feel bitter.

You remember Father Juan well, Olga, the priest who worked as a psychologist at Boscana. You used to amuse Father Juan with that sense of humour of yours, but one day you said something which astonished him. He told me about it because I wasn't there at the time. I don't know what feast-day it was, but he was going to give a talk to all the girls at Boscana, to preach a kind of sermon. He used to tell you from time to time to practise the Christian virtues, I suppose, and to talk to you about God, and say how you should love your parents and your brothers and sisters and the teachers . . .

That day, before he began his sermon and while he was chatting to you all, it occurred to you to say to him: "And now are you going to tell us the same things you usually do?" Father Juan explained to me that you had said it with a serene awareness of what you were saying, and that he didn't know what to answer and that he was still thinking about it the next day. That your simple remark had made him reflect a great deal, and led him to consider his choice of words, which perhaps had become rather routine.

Yes, I should like to have filled a notebook with all your odd jokes and with your simple truths, but I'm not sure really that by trying to evaluate all this expressive material I could really get to know you thoroughly.

And why should I understand you thoroughly if it's not possible to achieve this with anyone? I think that I know you up to a certain point, dear Olga, but all that I've been saying about you in these letters is a totally inadequate approximation to what you are.

We know what Down's Syndrome is, but we can't get anywhere near knowing what sort of individual any one of the Down's people is. Each has also been born with a personality which – like mine, like everyone's – is unique, indescribable, and which cannot be diagnosed by a computer. And as they have grown, in each one, we don't know how, alongside the invariable syndrome has developed their own internal world, not only through their congenital potentialities but also through the various environmental influences, which differ in each case.

And so, Olga, I love you for what I know of you and for what you give me, but I also love what you have of mystery, that innermost fortress of your thoughts and sentiments which in your "deficiency" cannot be reached by my "knowledge".

And I love this inability to know you completely, because it shows me that you're not a subproduct of nature that can be infallibly catalogued, but a fully human being. And it is precisely this complexity that defines a human being, a complexity that cannot be imprisoned within any codification or data bank.

17 WE'RE STILL TOGETHER

Dear Olga

I called you Olga in memory of a girl who died young. Younger than you are now.

When you were a little girl, several doctors gave their opinion that you probably wouldn't live long, that subnormal children tended to suffer certain illnesses against which they had very little defence. It was certainly so years ago, but nowadays there are many resources which help them to survive.

In your case it can only be said that your health is excellent, apart from specific anomalies such as defective teeth, short-sightedness and your lameness. But you don't really know what it means to feel ill. I can't remember how many years it is since I saw you in bed with an illness, not even with flu. Your systems function correctly, and although you have a congenital intestinal malfunction you eat a lot and digest it easily. So you are remarkably healthy, and you don't take any sort of medicine.

Is it likely that you'll go on having birthday after birthday and reach old age? Is it possible that your physical development is really the same as that of a normal adult?

Perhaps the idea that those who are mentally defective live less long makes it difficult for me to accept this, although at the age of thirty you are in the same physical state as most people of your age. I believe that that sudden collapse, that unpreventable injury or infection they prophesied, may happen at any moment. The truth is that I haven't wanted to consult any expert on what your expectation of life is – theoretically, I know – according to the most up-to-date knowledge. I don't want to be affected by any opinion which, like others, may turn out to be absolutely wrong.

So I sometimes ask myself, dear Olga, which of us two will die first, who will be the first to "go to heaven". This is the question which is usually the most heart-breaking one for parents. What will become of our subnormal children when we are no longer here?

I must be rather peculiar because usually I don't think about it, and I haven't made any decisions about trying to fill the probable financial and emotional void my absence might cause. I must be frank: I haven't planned anything to do with my personal future either, nor for the rest of the family. I've always had a trusting attitude towards life. Perhaps it's imprudent of me, but that's how it is, it must be a defect of my character. And this trust up to now has not been disappointed. I believe that valid solutions can always be found and that in the majority of cases the solutions don't depend on anything that we ourselves have presupposed.

Obviously I might die tomorrow. It's a possibility that doesn't worry me perhaps because I accepted the fact of death many years ago, quite naturally, I think. And the idea that you might survive me, Olga, doesn't cause me anxiety, as it reasonably might do. I have to tell you because it is so. I must be a reckless person, but I believe that your goodness will always find goodness, that your adaptability will always find someone who will adapt to you. But the money . . . Yes, money, obviously. But is it possible in this changing society to imagine that a financial decision taken now could still be effective in many years time, when you are seventy, say? Only up to a certain point, I think, and I'm not sure about that. I still base my faith on tomorrow's people rather than on tomorrow's money, and on the development of the social conscience. It's also true that I can't imagine you growing old. Perhaps it's because I have no experience, no visual image, of Down's girls becoming old ladies. Is it because they don't achieve it, as they say? Is it because they haven't achieved it yet because they are physically vulnerable but now, thanks to antibiotics and other remedies, they will grow old like everyone else? Will you perhaps be one of the first generation of Down's people to have a long life?

Sometimes I think that I don't want that to happen, and it's an idea that I don't very much want to turn over in my mind. For me you are a kind of angel who has somehow appeared in our lives and it seems consistent that some day or other you will abandon us unexpectedly too, and leave us with the memory of you as the great mystery of our existence.

Is it ridiculous of me to call you a sort of angel? I meant that you have never been a heavy burden, an obstacle in my path, a maggot nibbling away at my happiness. Quite the contrary, you have been and are a shining banner in the sea of my contradictions. Your death would not "take a load off my back" but would snatch from me the little bit of light that has never failed me. Obviously I could live without you, but I can't imagine it.

These are the last lines I shall write to you, dear Olga. Every day I've addressed a letter to you, often early in the morning when everyone was asleep, including you. I've enjoyed shutting myself up in my little study, listening to the silence and writing without stopping and without re-reading anything. I've done it in a strange haste, like someone drawing up an urgent, essential document, and I don't really know whether I was writing a will or a birth certificate for life.

Now it's done, and, as usual with everything I've written, I'll soon forget it.

There will be new jobs, new preoccupations, new books. And one day you'll announce to me, "There's football on the television." And we'll go and have lunch at the pizzeria, and they'll call you *signorinella*, and you'll open your eyes wide again and we'll see your kitten face better. And we'll never find you the ideal insoles, and some day or other in the car we'll sing the *piccolissima serenata* as we did so many years ago, "which can be sung with a thin voice", *un filo di voce*.

With your thin little voice, dear Olga, we've sung the song of life.

With kisses, as always, up to ten: as I gave you the ten kisses, you learned to count. And you – tender and full of fun – have always liked to respond with eleven.

Thank you for everything, dear Olga.